HOW I LOST 40 POUNDS WHILE ENJOYING BEEF, BUTTER, AND BORDEAUX

And How You Can, Too

CADE CONNORS

This book is not intended to substitute for the consultation, diagnosis and/or medical treatment of your own physician or healthcare provider.

INTRODUCTION

Hi, my name is Cade Connors, and I was a chunk, a butterball, a flabmeister. Also a pretty successful lawyer, the corporate kind, who spent a lot of time on his butt in a chair.

At fifty-five, I looked at myself sideways in the mirror and saw the profile of Alfred Hitchcock.

"Time to drop some pounds," I said.

"What did you just say?" My wife was walking past the bathroom.

"I'm going to lose some weight!"

"You've been saying that for years."

"This time I mean it."

The lovely Sue came into the bathroom. "I hope you're serious this time," she said. "We've been down this road before."

Yes, down that long, winding road.

When we got married, I was a Greek god. I don't mind saying it. I'd been a varsity athlete in high school and college. I'd put on a few pounds by the time I met Sue, but my chiseled form was still apparent under a tight T-shirt. Plus, I had all my hair.

A couple of years after the wedding, our first child was born. We planned to have more, but our income was light. That's when I decided to go to law school.

Ah, those days and nights on my caboose in the classroom and library. And with easy access to campus fast food and vending machines.

The pounds started ticking upward.

Then came professional life, the stress of a young lawyer trying to make good. My favorite way to deal with stress was with food. Wonderful, comforting carbs. The siren song of sugar.

Two more children came along.

When the last of our brood went off to college, I was fifty pounds over my wedding weight.

Several times my wife suggested I try a diet program. I always huffed it off. She didn't nag me about it, and when she prepped a meal it was always a balanced one. But I did a lot of my eating out, especially lunches near the office. The pot stayed on me like an unwelcome alien sucking the life out of its host..

I finally agreed to try Weight Watchers.

I've got nothing against WW. But for me, trying to eat what they suggested was like chomping varieties of cardboard. I know that's harsh; it's just what it felt like. I did earn a five-pound ribbon, and that was great. But I stalled out. I didn't want to eat that way the rest of my life.

So let's cut back to the scene of me and the mirror and the missus. I was now sixty, count 'em, sixty pounds over my wedding weight.

Now what?

Was I fated to some draconian diet plan? Liposuction? Freezing the fat? Moving to Devil's Island for the summer?

A friend of mine who topped the scales at 300 plus went on a plan with a nutritionist. It was miraculous. He shed 110 pounds in what seemed like record time. His skin, however, was having a hard time adjusting. You could pack a lunch in the sags around his neck. Still, he had dropped all those awful LBs!

I almost joined him. But I just wasn't ready for apple slices and a diet shake plan.

A year later, I saw this friend again, and he had gained almost all the weight back!

I began to feel hopeless. I went around quoting Victor Buono fat poems. Like his prayer:

"You are what you eat," said a wise old man.
Lord, if that's true, I'm a garbage can!
I want to rise on judgment day, that's plain;
But at my present weight, I'll need a crane.

And, Lord, I pray with folded pinkies,
Deliver me from Hostess Twinkies.
And when my time of trial is done
And my war with malted milks is won,
Let me stand with the saints in heaven
In a shining robe size thirty-seven.

I finally decided to do some research and figure out how to dump some serious blubber. Along the way I learned, ahem, an inconvenient truth: what the government has been handing us about nutrition for the last 60 years has hurt more people than it has helped. We're fatter than ever!

To cut to the end point, I dropped forty pounds and

have stayed in that zone for almost two years. I expect to stay here the rest of my life.

In this little book, I'll tell you how it happened.

Hint: It wasn't hard at all.

Now, I must wrap up this introduction with the obligatory legal disclaimer. I'm a lawyer, after all, but not a doctor or a licensed health professional. Nor have I ever played either one on TV. So what is in this book is not professional advice. Any steps you take should be talked over with your own doc or nutritionist. This book is not intended to substitute for the consultation, diagnosis and/or medical treatment of your own physician or healthcare provider.

I do encourage you to do your own research so that, when you talk things over with your professional, you're an informed yakker and not some schlub who blindly does whatever anybody tells him. We have too many such citizens today. They forget that the founders of our great nation were tired of getting led around by the nose by a distant monarch. They laid out their case in the Declaration of Independence, stating: *The history of the present King of Great Britain is a history of repeated injuries and usurpations, all having in direct object the establishment of an absolute Tyranny over these States. To prove this, let Facts be submitted to a candid world.*

So here in this book, I submit my facts.

Bon appétit!

WHAT WE ALL THOUGHT WAS TRUE IS NOT

Diets. All kinds of diets are out there. And most of them work—if you work them—for a while.

Problem is, most people fall off the wagon at some point.

Most diets have meal plans, but I could never stick to those. I want spontaneity! If I was supposed to have broiled fish but my mouth was shouting for a steak, I wanted the meat. (I'm a lawyer. I can't disrespect my mouth.)

Also, the diets were not favorable about alcohol. Now, there are abundant reasons to be careful when discussing distilled spirits. Last thing we need is more alcoholics. But I like a civilized drink in the evening. (See "The Bourdeaux Part" up ahead).

The whole matter came into focus one day when one of my law partners made a joke at lunch. As he dipped another onion ring in ranch dressing, he looked at me and said, "You know, scientists have confirmed that if you eat healthy, you won't live longer. It'll just seem longer."

Made perfect sense to me.

But at what cost? We've been warned, over and over again, about heart disease and its enabler, cholesterol.

So, almost as a lark, I did some study. And something I found stunned me: When our government started laying down dietary guidelines, in the late 1970s, the average American man weighed 170 pounds.

The average Joe now tips the scales at 197! (Women went from 145 to 170.)

During that same period, child obesity became a massive crisis. And Type 2 diabetes has gone from 2% to 10% in this land of dietary guidelines.

Good work, federal government! What the heck?

THE IKE SPIKE

How did we get to this dismal state of affairs? It appears to have started with the "Ike Spike."

Ike was the nickname of President Dwight D. Eisenhower. When he suffered a heart attack while in office, it got the country's attention. What do we do about this? What experts can help us solve this national menace?

Remember, this was in the 1950s, when medical science and science in general were exploding with advancements, like putting men into space and curing terrible diseases. Polio was conquered by Dr. Jonas Salk, who became a hero.

That kind of fame is catnip to the ambitious—which is not necessarily a bad thing. It can motivate someone to press further on in scientific or medical research. But it can also lead to the lust for fame. Scientists are not immune to the human condition. Sometimes, then, the more persuasive or charismatic figure might carry the day, and gather around him a populist army to defend his battlements.

That appears to be what happened when a researcher from the University of Minnesota, Ancel Keys, delivered what he called a "Seven Countries Study" purporting to prove that people who consumed high amounts of fat—specifically, saturated fat—had higher cholesterol levels and thus, higher rates of heart attacks. So all you have to do is eat less fat!

The bandwagon formed and everyone jumped on. Well, almost everyone. But the ones who didn't, who said, "Maybe we should do a little more study before we tell everybody in the country how to eat," they got muzzled.

According to cardiologist Dr. Bret Scher:

> When other scientists questioned Keyes's conclusions, they were invariably met with stern responses like: "people are dying while you're quibbling over data points."[1]

Does that not sound familiar? (**cough** Covid **cough**)

Then along came the "food pyramid." All the little boys and girls at school, and their parents, had this visual drummed into their heads.

Only, ahem, we started getting fatter. Maybe not as fat as if we'd been given Dr. Nick Riviera's nutritional pyramid (Dr. Nick is a character from *The Simpsons.* He is a graduate of Hollywood Upstairs Medical School). His pyramid looked like this:

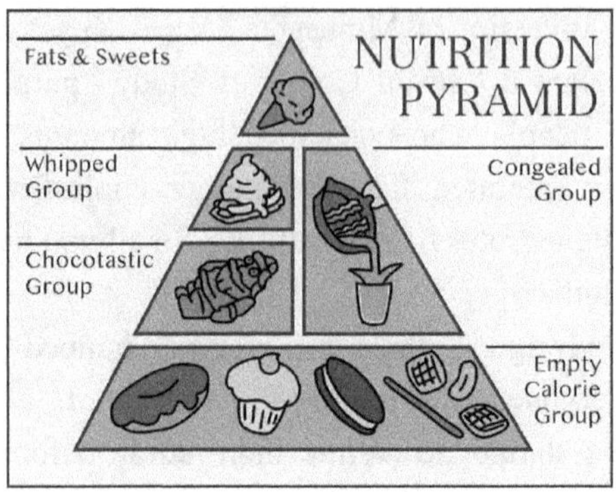

More from Dr. Sher:

As Americans ate less saturated fat—margarine instead of butter, processed oils like corn oil instead of olive oil, low fat milk, low fat yogurt and so on— they also started to eat more "heart healthy" grains—exactly what the food pyramid, and the updated version called MyPlate, advise you to do.

As the consumption of saturated fat decreased by almost 40%, the consumption of refined grains—carbohydrates that convert to sugar in the body—increased substantially. Total intake of calories also began to increase.

This happened, in no small part, because food companies took advantage of the low-fat craze. They lowered fat and increased sugar. Suddenly, supermarkets were full of supposedly healthy low fat, high-sugar foods. It remains that way today. Foods that are high in sugar stimulate reward centers in the brain and leave us wanting more. Thus, the famous line about potato chips: "Betcha can't eat just one!"

WHAT'S THE DEAL WITH CHOLESTEROL?

And then there was the demonization of cholesterol. This waxy, fat-like substance in our cells does a lot of work, like make hormones. Hormones are the Pony Express of your body. They carry messages through your blood to your organs, muscles and other tissues. These messages instruct your body—including the brain—how to function..

Now, for decades we've been told that it's the lowering of your cholesterol that is the key to preventing heart attacks. That has led to the statin boom. And to the bromide that it's fat that makes you fat.

But what if lowering LDL cholesterol is not the key to heart health? Indeed, what if brain function is adversely affected *because of* reduced cholesterol via statins?

At least it's something to think about, so long as we are allowed to think at all (a freedom that has come under serious attack lately, considering all the "deplatforming" going on when doctors dare to question "the science.")

IT'S THE CLOTS, DUDE

In his book *The Clot Thickens* (what a great title!) Dr. Malcolm Kendrick makes the case for "the thrombogenic hypothesis." *Thrombo* is short for thrombosis, which is the formation of a blood clot (known as a thrombus) within a blood vessel. *Genesis*, of course, means the creation of something, as in the heavens and the earth (Genesis 1:1)...or heart disease.

This is not a new theory, by the way. All the way back in 1852 a Viennese doctor named Carl von Rokitansky noticed "encrustation" in the blood vessels of certain dead people (he was an autopsy guy, among other things). The good doctor posited that when a blood clot forms on the arterial wall, normally it will dissolve. That's called "repair." But if repair doesn't happen fast enough, and another clot starts to form in the same general area, it results in what is called *atherosclerotic plaque.*

So, under this hypothesis, plaque is not the collected, piled-up goo from cholesterol. It's unrepaired blood clots.

According to Dr. Kendrick: "We know blood clots cause the final event in cardiovascular disease. We know blood clots cause plaques to grow. Why won't we accept that blood clots are the thing that starts heart disease in the first place? Because then we have one process all the way through, and it makes sense, because it fits with what you can see."

Now, if you want to get more into this I recommend Dr. Kendrick's book. For our purposes, I'm just trying to point out that not every expert believes cholesterol is the villain in our heart's melodrama.

For one more note on this, see this report titled "Inflammation, not Cholesterol, Is a Cause of Chronic Disease."[2] The abstract states:

> In this review, we present all the relevant data that supports the view that it is inflammation induced by several factors, such as platelet-activating factor (PAF), that leads to the onset of cardiovascular diseases (CVD) rather than serum cholesterol. The key to reducing the incidence of CVD is to control the activities of PAF and other inflammatory mediators via diet, exercise, and healthy lifestyle choices. The relevant studies and data supporting these views are discussed in this review.

SO HOW DID I LOSE WEIGHT?

So, how did I start losing weight?

I'm glad you asked.

I did not find a diet. My diet found me. *Not*, I quickly add, a "diet plan." Just how I eat.

Here's what happened.

In the early stages of the WuFlu, when everyone was going batty trying to figure out what to do—and no, I don't use "batty" to refer to the theory that this pestilence came from a bat sold in a Chinese wet market—I mean nutty, which I don't find fault with, because we hadn't faced anything like this before, at least not in our lifetime, at least not since the 1918 flu epidemic that killed millions.

The panic mode was understandable, and so was fear. *To a point.*

So from on high, and before the so-called "vaccine" (which turned out not to be a vaccine, because vaccines prevent, or at least used to until the CDC changed the definition to fit the data) the powers that be decided that if we locked down and wore masks for 15 days we could "slow the spread."

How'd that turn out?

You know how. You know that the nationwide lockdowns were a disaster, leading to spikes in suicide, spousal abuse, drug overdoses, children falling behind in school, and small business dropping like flies in a fumigated house.

So many restaurants suffered, collapsed, and died. Especially here in L.A., where the varied cuisines are the envy of the world.

It was during this time, when my wife and I stopped going out to eat, that my lard started to melt.

I looked at the scale one day and saw that I was ten pounds lighter. How in the heck did that happen?

The answer came to me—I was eating a whole lot less bread. Every time my wife and I went out to eat, they served bread. Every hamburger and hot dog I grabbed for lunch had bread. My go-to lunch beverage at the time, beer, is liquid bread. Just by cutting down on those things I was getting rid of a whole lot of bad carbs.

And sugar. I love apple fritters. I'd indulge myself at least once a week. Sheepishly, I admit I didn't often share this information with my wife. Ditto the scones with my Starbucks.

Now I wasn't getting these nearly so often.

With restaurants closed, we naturally cooked more at home. We ate steaks, eggs, fish, and figured out some great ways to cook greens, like Brussels Sprouts and broccoli (yes, broccoli, steamed and with *butter*.)

A couple more months and I was down twenty pounds.

Not to say we didn't eat some bread or have a piece of pie now and then. Just a lot less of both.

And whenever I did get an apple fritter, I discovered I no longer wanted the whole thing. I found that if I ate half or a quarter of it I felt fine and satisfied. And had a nice treat left over to split with my wife over morning coffee.

I still enjoyed a civilized evening cocktail. Usually a martini or bourbon rocks—and a little research had told me these have zero carbs.

I remembered a little book that caused a sensation in the 1960s called *The Drinking Man's Diet.* My dad had it. I even remembered a joke Red Skelton told on his TV show. Dean Martin, of course, had a rep as a big drinker, so Red said Dean was on the Drinking Man's Diet. "Now he weighs 94 pounds!"

The little booklet sold 2.4 million copies back in the mid-60s. Then some Harvard medical guy came out with a big warning that this diet was "mass murder."

Sales dried up immediately, as the medical profession convinced everyone this low-carb diet was a ticking time bomb.

A little research took me to an article in *Forbes* that profiled the author of the book, Gardner Jameson. Guess what? He was still kicking it at the age of 93! And still enjoying his cocktails.

What was his secret?

Just eat under 60 grams of carbs a day. And most liquor has no carbs.

I jumped at this.

The months went by, and in L.A. they kept up the lock-downs and mask craziness longer than any other city. When it was deemed okay to go to a restaurant, provided you wore a mask (except when you ate, because the virus was polite and did not spread while you chomped) we still chose to stay mostly at home and cook for ourselves.

But we did not remain house bound. We wanted fresh air, so began taking walks. In those days, we'd see so many folks walking alone, outside on a sunny day, masked up! On more than one occasion we'd be walking toward a masked peripatetic who would spot our faces and, I'm not kidding, cross the street to the other side!

Cutting to the proverbial chase, after about eight months, I stepped on the scale and saw I was down 40 pounds!

I felt comfortable and serene. Old pants fit again. I had more energy. So I've made it my goal to remain in the zone between 215 and 220 for the rest of my life.

The only thing I think about is carbs (not including fruits and veggies). I try to eat under 60 grams of carbs a day. I used to use an app that keeps track of the carbs. But now I sort of have it in my head. A soft alarm goes off in my brain if I'm getting close to 60, and I'll just spend the rest of the day avoiding them.

Now, there's a bit more to what I did to lose those 40 pounds and how I've stayed in that zone, feeling good. I'll get to those things in a moment.

For now I just want to stress how easy it is to eat this way, because it makes you happy and will let you—if this is your desire—enjoy beef, butter, and Bordeaux.

Let's talk about each.

THE BEEF PART

Let's talk about meat.

I want you to know this is not a knock on vegans. There are those for whom this is the path, for a variety of reasons, some health related, some philosophy related, or a mix of the two. If that's you, fine and dandy. I'm only presenting my view in this book. I have long believed that if God did not want us to eat cows, he would not have made them of meat. A good steak is proof that God exists and wants us to be happy.

It also happens that beef is an excellent source of protein (and in my humble opinion, the best). Beef is also a terrific source of iron. According to WebMd: "The iron in beef helps your body produce hemoglobin, a protein that helps your blood carry oxygen from your lungs to the rest of your body."[1] If your iron intake is deficient, you can get tired, lazy, listless, and brain foggy.

Beef delivers zinc, too, which we all know from the Covid scourge is essential for the immune system. Here's an interesting note in that regard.

Do you know why the old advice "An apple a day keeps the doctor away" works?

It's because of the quercetin in the apples. Quercetin is an ionophore. What that does is help zinc (which you find in abundance in meat and eggs) get into the cells. So the people of old who ate apples and meat and eggs were building up strong immune systems, thus keeping the doctor away!

When Covid hit and some doctors said, "Hey! This FDA-approved drug called Hydroxychloroquine seems to be working to prevent and heal Covid" it was because HQC is an ionophore, too, and with a zinc supplement the cells become a Spartan army to fight off viruses.

(One of the great scandals in medical history is the demonization of HQC. History will not be kind to the "health experts" who consigned thousands to death or hospitalization because of this ban.)

Include fruits and vegetables in your eating, for sure. I've read about folks who've done an all-meat diet and feel better than ever. I don't know enough about that to say yea or nay. I only know that I like to eat apples for snacks. And celery sticks. And baked Brussels sprouts. Spinach salad.

The eating of meat will not make you fat. Indeed, meat is packed with fats that are actually good for your heart. (Ack! Can you hear the wailing and gnashing of teeth out there? If so, I recommend Bose Noise Cancelling headphones.)

It is true that meat *products* like sausage, ham, salami, hot dogs and cured meats have high levels of sodium. The answer here is, don't eat a lot of those, but on occasion, enjoy! One of my favorite snacks (the key word is *snacks*) is pepperoni slices. Every three months or so I have to have a good ol' hot dog—in a bun, of course—with mustard and diced onions (or sauerkraut).

But for a main course, give me steak. Especially a ribeye.

I like 'em cooked two ways.

One is on the grill. The other is in a cast-iron skillet.

Use a choice or prime cut. Some people like bone-in, but I don't sense a real flavor difference. My wife and I prefer boneless cuts, cooked medium rare.

We prep the meat with McCormick Montreal Steak Seasoning. The rub is up to you, of course. Some Kosher salt and fresh ground pepper works just fine. Put these in a bowl and dole it out with your fingers. Sprinkle generously on all sides, including the edges. Let the meat sit for five minutes to soak in.

For grilling, heat your grill to 350°. Put on the meat. After five minutes, flip the meat over. To know when it's done, you can use the "poke test" with your finger. It should feel like when you press your finger into the base of your thumb.

But I prefer a good meat thermometer. I aim for 135° internal temperature. Then take off the meat and let it sit for five minutes.

With a cast-iron skillet, my preferred method is as follows.

Season the meat as above. Heat your oven to 350°.

Set the skillet on high heat with a coating of avocado oil. When the skillet is good and hot, put on the steak let it sear for two minutes. Flip it and sear for another two minutes. Then put the skillet in the oven and cook to an internal temp of 135°.

I sometimes add a few cloves of garlic in the skillet before putting on the meat.

Let the meat rest. Then eat it.

Experiment with different cuts of beef. You can find abundant recipes on the internet. Chicken and pork chops are also part of my culinary intake. But when it comes right down to it, I prefer the cow.

Eat fish from time to time. Salmon is good for the brain. White fish fights inflammation and strengthens your immune system.

Have fun with all this. Stay away from processed foods and copious amounts of sugar, except on rare occasions. A Twinkie on the Fourth of July is not going to hurt you. A bit of natural sugar in your coffee, with a dollop of cream, is fine—though when you develop a taste for black coffee, you'll find you don't really need it.

Don't worry if you blast over your carb count one day. Just don't make it every day.

Try eating half of something sweet next time. Instead of a thick piece of pie, go for a sliver. Make a habit of it and you'll find you're satisfied with less. Sugar bombing will make you lousy. Good!

Oh yes, water. You need to drink it, though you don't have to drown yourself. Have a small glass first thing in the morning. Drink several cups throughout the day, and you're golden.

A final note. Your grandmother (or great grandmother for you kids) was right about the importance of a good ol' bowel movement each day. Try for a grunty in the morning. A glass of water and cup of coffee helps me in this regard.

You're welcome!

THE BUTTER PART

I have a vivid memory from my childhood. I was around 8 or 9, at a community event with my parents. We sat at a table with some other families.

Next to me was a kid around 12, on the chunky side. He set about to butter a roll. But before he could lay the spread on the bread, his mother grabbed his hand and took away the knife.

"People get heart attacks!" she said.

The poor lad got a pained expression on his face, which I could read as if it were in neon: AWW, MOM!

But this was at the height of the new government attack on fat.

And as I grew up, the danger of butter became calcified as "common knowledge."

This "knowledge" resulted in another fad: oleomargarine. Butter substitutes. The most famous of these products was called I Can't Believe It's Not Butter. Another was Chiffon Soft Stick Margarine. There was a commercial on TV about it. A woman in the woods, Mother Nature, has a taste of her "sweet, creamy butter." So good!

The narrator informs her it is not butter at all, but this new product. "Chiffon fooled you."

She wags her finger. "It's not nice to fool Mother Nature!" Suddenly there's the crash of thunder and the woods are laid waste! The jingle went, "If you think it's butter, but it's not, it's Chiffon!"

Problem is, margarine goes through a process called hydrogenation, which adds hydrogen to the oil. That creates "trans fat" which ain't good for you.

And listen to what WebMD says: "In moderation, butter can be a healthy part of your diet. It's rich in nutrients like bone-building calcium and contains compounds linked to lower chances of obesity."[1]

Whoa! If I could only go back in time and tell that mom that her kid would be better off with butter on that roll!

There's more. Butter is high in beta-carotene, which your body converts to Vitamin A. And beta-carotene has been linked to lowered risks of lung cancer and prostate cancer.

Double wow!

Beta-carotene may help slow the rate of vision loss and age-related macular degeneration. It helps your bones avoid osteoporosis. Butter has Vitamin E, great for your skin.

Use up more wows here!

Now, of course, you don't go around eating sticks of butter—except at the Iowa State Fair that serves deep fried butter on a stick (once in a lifetime is enough for that).

But moderate use of butter for cooking and spreading is a good thing and won't make you fat.

A WORD ON INTERMITTENT FASTING

You want to burn fat even though you eat fat?

Intermittent fasting is something you might consider.

Relax, it's not ascetic fasting, like a monk. You don't have to wear camel's hair and rest between meals of locusts and wild honey.

All it means is you eat your meals within an 8-hour window.

So you can have your breakfast at 9 and finish dinner at 5. Or breakfast at 10 and finish eating at 6.

When I first tried this, my stomach really growled at me in the morning. I didn't give up my morning coffee, black. But I didn't eat. After a couple of days it became easier to wait until 9 or 10.

What happens when you fast is that your body has a chance to break down the sugar in your body (called glycogen stores). When that's gone, your body starts burning fat.

Nice deal.

THE BORDEAUX PART

Right up until his death at the age of 100, comedian George Burns was still sharp and funny. "Every morning I wake up and read the obituaries," he quipped. "If my name's not there I have breakfast."

Once, when he was 96, he went on a talk show, smoking his ever-present cigar. When the host questioned him on this, Burns said he smoked fifteen cigars a day and had a martini in the evening.

"What does your doctor say about that?" the host asked.

"My doctor's dead," Burns said.

Which brings me to a few words about drinking.

Moderate drinking will not make you fat.

Now, we all know alcoholism and drug addiction are very, very bad. And that some people are more predisposed by genetics to an addictive profile.

We also know there are various complicating factors, including how early someone starts to drink or drug.

So I'm not going to advocate that you start drinking. I am simply going to tell you that drinking in moderation—if such is possible for you—will not make you fat.

There are a couple of provisos, however. First of all, beer is full of carbohydrates, so be aware of that. Second, adding sugary mixtures to spirits will drive up the carb count.

That said, I do enjoy a civilized martini and a fine Bordeaux. If you'll indulge me, just a few words on these libations.

CIVILIZED MARTINI

By civilized martini, I mean a base of 3 oz. of *gin*. In the good old days, when you ordered a martini, gin is what you'd get. Then along came Ian Fleming and James Bond drinking *vodka* martinis. Now many folks think this is the only real martini. Oh, the humanity!

Gin is the real deal.

A martini is—get ready—gin and vermouth.

How much vermouth? That's entirely up to you. Experiment with it. A dry martini has very little vermouth. The driest martini is the kind Winston Churchill drank. He would pour the gin and look at the vermouth bottle across the room. (And I'll remind you, he's the guy who saved Western Civilization.)

A classic martini also has a stuffed olive in it. You can play around with this. My mom liked a pearl onion, which turns the martini into a Gibson (which is what Cary Grant and Eva Marie Saint drink on the train in *North by Northwest*. You can't get classier than that!)

With more complex botanical gins (like Hendrick's) I prefer a lemon twist.

If you choose to have a martini, let me give you some humorous—yet serious—advice from the writer James Thurber: "One martini is all right. Two are too many, and three are not enough." (If you watched the TV series *Mad Men*, you know exactly what this means.)

BORDEAUX

I don't have to tell you the benefits of red wine. Ever since *60 Minutes* did a report called "The French Paradox" the medical journals have been all over it. Back in 1991, reporter Morley Safer sat down at a bistro in Lyon, France and started talking about all the fat, butter, and oil in the French diet. He then asked why it was that the French have less heart disease than the low-fat crazed Americans.

He lifted a glass of red wine, and said, "The answer to the riddle, the explanation of the paradox, may lie in this inviting glass."[1]

The theory, he explained, was that red wine has a way of cleansing the arteries.

Boom! Americans started going gaga for red wine.

Red wine has antioxidants called polyphenols that help protect the lining of blood vessels in the heart. One of these polyphenols is called resveratrol, which seems to protect blood vessels *and* prevent blood clots. Nice!

So when I have a steak I want a good glass of red with it.

Of course, the "medical profession" is reserved on resveratrol, and reticent on a good red. The American Heart Association says the benefits of red wine can also be obtained through fruits and vegetables.

To the AHA, I offer this little poem:

God in his goodness gave us the grape
To please both great and small.

Little fools will drink too much;
Great fools none at all.

THE EXERCISE AND MUSCLE PART (WHICH YOU'LL LOVE)

You want to be a lean, mean muscled machine? I don't mean pumped up like Arnold on steroids (which is redundant). I mean be healthy and strong for your age.

You can do it without weights or gym memberships or hours

You know how that goes. You get serious about working out. You go down and buy a gym membership. The first month you kill it. Three or four times a week. You work up a good sweat. Push weights or machines. Get that treadmill heated up. Heck, you do 20 minutes at level 4. Nice going!

But then you start to taper off. It's hard to get ready and then drive 10, 15, 20 minutes to the gym. You suit up, exercise, shower, get dressed, come home. An hour-and-a-half out of your day.

Pretty soon, you're saying "Nah" more often.

But we all know it's important to be in good physical shape. If only there was a way to do that in mere minutes, without leaving the house. And without having to change into gym clothes.

Well, I'm here to tell you, there is such a way.

If you're a lard lad or lass, and hate the idea of exercising for 20 or 30 minutes a throw, then give yourself 30 seconds. Can you manage 30 seconds of moving fast?

Here's the deal on that. There's been studies on what's called High Impact Interval Training (HIIT) that say short, intense workouts—which can easily be done at home—will burn more fat than half an hour on a treadmill.

HIIT works better at burning fat because it revs up the metabolism, as opposed to aerobics, which is cardio. With HIIT you also continue to burn fat *after* the workout. This post-workout effect can last up to 72 hours!

But it's really the time element I like. As reported on the Penn Medicine News website:

> "Interval training has gained interest lately because research has suggested that you make similar gains in cardiovascular fitness as you would with traditional endurance exercise regimens, but with shorter periods of exercise," said Neel Chokshi, MD, MBA, director of Penn's Sports Cardiology & Fitness Program. "So, if you do not have time for the traditionally recommended 150 minutes of moderate intensity exercise each week, this may serve as a substitute. The 'better' exercise regimen is arguably the one that is consistent and sustainable to see gains over time."[1]

At a basic level, HIIT means working intense for 30 seconds, easing off a bit (but not stopping) for 30, then doing 30 more hard, 30 off and so on...for only four minutes!

Doesn't that beat driving to an expensive club, sweating

hard for an hour, showering and dressing and driving back home and boom...two hours of your day are gone?

Hard as it is to believe, you can get good, healthy results in just four minutes in your bedroom. And not even every day. Three or four days a week of this is optimum.

MY WORKOUT

HIIT is clinical sounding. I call my workout "Stick-and-move."

The term stick-and-move comes from the world of boxing. It means moving your feet as you jab, jab, jab your opponent, setting him up for the knockout blow.

My stick-and-move workout is me basically shadow boxing. You move both legs and arms. I like to do this in front of a full-length mirror and put the hurt on my own reflection.

I use an interval timer app, set for eight 30-second intervals. It starts beeping 3-2-1 at the end of each interval.

I stick-and-move for 30 seconds.

I then do slow walking, swinging my arms easily, for 30.

Then 30 more of stick-and-move, 30 slow-walk, and so on till the end.

So you have four intervals of stick-and-move, where you get your heart rate up. You want to get to a place where it's a little hard to have a conversation.

The slow-walk times give you a bit of a rest, while still keeping the ticker going.

What's great about this routine is that you control how intense it is. If you're getting too out of breath, you just slow down what you're doing. If you're not out of breath enough, pick up the pace.

I mix up my punches, too. Mostly jabs with each arm, but also straight punches, upper cuts, body shots. Sometimes I just twirl my fists in front of my chest.

And move those feet, always move them. You can shuffle, hop, run in place. You can even slow walk as long as you're vigorously moving your arms. The arms are really the key to getting the most out of this routine.

After the four minutes, walk softly in place for a minute to wind down. Then do some stretching for 2–3 minutes. Then a minute or two of deep breathing—in through the nose, hold, then out slowly through pursed lips.

And you're done! Not only will you be getting heart healthy, you'll drop pounds.

How can this be?

Apparently this type of workout gets your metabolism churning longer and more efficiently than a medium effort, thirty-minute aerobic workout. I don't know why that is, but it is.

Some days, I might just do a few 30-second walks through the house, moving my arms like a paddle-wheel motion in front of my chest.

Now, get this. The effects of a 30 second, heart-pumping don't have to be consecutive. They are also cumulative.

That is, if I shadow box for 30 seconds, then wind down for 30, I can stop...and do another round an hour later. And the effect is the same.

Think about that. Can you do 30 seconds? Yes! I'd say you can do that in your sleep, but then I'd be advocating pugilistic somnambulism. I don't want you punching your significant other.

So let me tell you what I do sometimes. I'm at one end of my house and I need to go to the other end. I'll do a shuffle step, sort of a slow jog, while spinning my arms in front of me. When I get to the other side, I'm winded. Nice!

Then I do some "get-ups." If I've been sitting watching a movie or TV show, I just get up, keep watching, and do "stepping jacks" for 30 seconds. I walk in place and flap my arms up and down (as in a traditional jumping jack).

You can increase the intensity by lifting your legs a little higher and stepping a little faster.

Same thing when I've been at my desk working on the computer. Every half hour I get up and do my routine for 30 seconds.

STRENGTH TRAINING

Keeping your muscles in shape is really important, especially as we get older. It's necessary for the bones, the metabolism, even the brain. Yes, being toned helps you think better, and may be one of the key methods for staving off dementia.

You don't need fancy weights or machines to keep your muscles in good shape. If you're young and you want to look like a Greek god or goddess, and push weights for mass, that's fine.

But most of us don't have the time for that. We want to be lean and taut.

Once again, you don't need a ton of time to get this way.

Use my 30-Second method and concentrate on your arms, tummy, and legs.

Actually, let me give credit where credit is due. I owe this to Charles Atlas.

Maybe you've never heard of him, but if you were a boy in the 1950s or 60s who read comic books you sure did. On the back cover of many a Superman or Batman comic was a six-panel cartoon strip that told a story.

The title of the story was "The Insult That Made a Man Out of Mac."

A rather skinny lad (Mac) is sitting on a beach with a nicely appointed lass. A muscled guy runs by, kicking up sand in their faces. "Hey!" Mac says. "Quit kicking sand in our faces!" The girl remarks, "That man is the worst nuisance on the beach."

The bully pulls Mac up and says, "Listen here. I'd smash your face—only you're so skinny you might dry up and blow away."

When he leaves, Mac says, "The big bully! I'll get even some day."

But the gal snipes, "Oh, don't let it bother you, little boy."

Sheesh! This was the dance of romance back then.

Back in his room, Mac kicks over a chair. He's looking at a magazine ad and says, "Darn it! I'm sick and tired of being a scarecrow! Charles Atlas says he can give me a REAL body, all right! I'll gamble a stamp and get his FREE book!"

The next panel says LATER...how much later we're not told, but hey, this is a short comic strip. Mac is standing in front of his mirror and he is bulked up and ripped! "Boy! It didn't take Atlas long to do this for me! That bully won't shove ME around again!"

In the next panel he's back at the beach with his girl. The bully has shown up. Mac says, "What! You here again? Here's something I owe you!" as he delivers a right to the guy's chin.

The end of the story shows the girl clinging to Mac. "Oh, Mac! You ARE a man after all!" Above them it says,

"Hero of the Beach." Another couple is looking at him. The girl says, "Gosh! What a build." The boy says, "He's already famous for it."

Next to that is a picture of Charles Atlas himself, once declared "The World's Most Perfectly Developed Man." The ad copy asks if you are "fed up with seeing the huskies walk off with the best of everything? Sick and tired of being soft, frail, skinny or flabby—only HALF ALIVE? I know just how you feel. Because I myself was once a puny 97-pound runt."

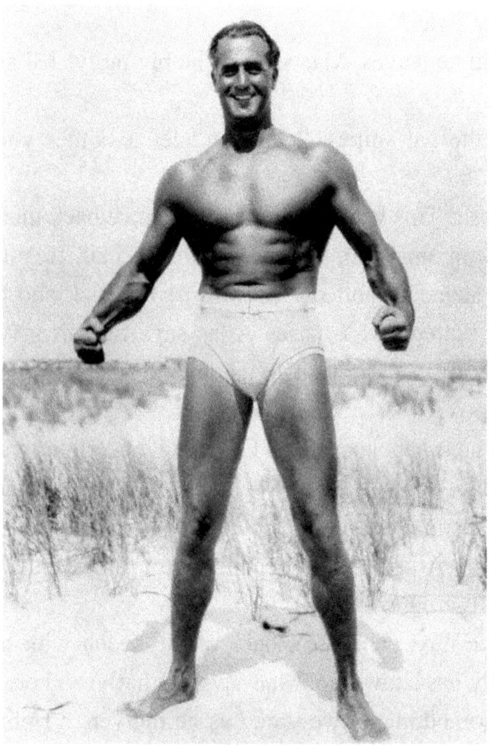

Charles Atlas

He tells how he discovered a wonderful way to develop his body FAST. He called his method Dynamic-Tension.

(Actually, the term was coined by a smart ad man named Charles Roman, who became Atlas's partner and made him a millionaire.)

The course he sold was a sensation. Some famous heavyweight boxers extolled its virtues, including Max Baer and the best of them all, Rocky Marciano.

Atlas followed his plan all his life, and it showed. His daily morning routine was 100 sit-ups, 300 pushups, and 50 knee bends.

I wanted to buy the course but my mom put the kibosh on that. When I was in my thirties I bought the course, and loved it. There's a lot in it about healthy eating—meat is primary!—and things like deep breathing, sunshine, a "music bath" and so on. I put it in a notebook and on my shelf. Where it stayed until I started losing weight and wanted to tone my bod.

Dynamic-Tension is isometrics, which is "pitting one muscle against another" for 6 seconds. You can work your arms this way in a variety of moves.

For instance, you cock on arm and put the fist of your other hand in the palm. You then push with the fist as you resist with the arm, for 6 seconds. I let the arm slowly go down. That works your triceps.

You can start the same way, only curling your arm up. That's for your biceps.

You can put your arms in front of your chest and push hard, working your lats.

You can do this anytime, anywhere.

There's also the good old push-up. Atlas would do his between two chairs. Man, that really works! At my age, though, I do push-ups from my knees. I do a set of about

20, rest, and do 20 more. Do what you can but stop before it becomes a strain. Find out what works for you, and you can build up from there.

If you're young and you want to get buff this way, you can do it. You don't need weights. Charles Atlas did it by doing 200 push-ups a day, in sets of 25. Work your way up slowly. Get to where you can do 25, rest for a bit, and do 25 more, rest, etc. Heck, you can watch TV while you do this.

Be sure to eat plenty of protein, especially the meat kind.

THE BACK AND TUMMY

Our core, made up of back and tummy muscles, can also be strengthened with Dynamic Tension.

Back

Sit in a chair with your back straight and feet on the ground. Move your lower back forward a bit and tighten those muscles. It takes a little practice, but you can do it. Hold that tightening for 7 seconds.

You can learn to do this standing, too

Tummy

Same chair position as in the above. Pull your tummy muscles in and tense them for 7 seconds.

You can do this standing or walking, too. Anytime!

The cumulative effect of all this is amazing for tone and bone. No weights. No gym.

I do crunches and squats, too. I do these on alternate days. The other days I do my high boxing routine. I take Sundays off.

That's really all you need, but I do want to take a moment to extol the benefits of an optional piece of equipment.

TOTAL GYM

I don't get any money from the Total Gym folks. When I saw Chuck Norris, looking fab in his 70s, endorsing this, I got one. It is cool as all get out. You use it for resistance training, similar to isometrics, with your body weight as counter balance. A routine is not time consuming, and once again I'm not going to a gym, just to my garage.

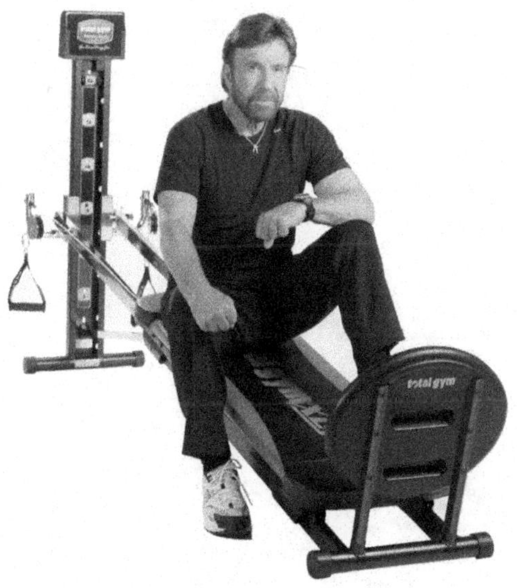

Chuck Norris. When he does a pushup, he's pushing the Earth down.

You can get one for yourself and there are hundreds of exercises you can do with this. I do only a few. One of my favorites is the reverse curl. Another is the push out.

I love it when another oldster slaps me on the arm to say hello or goodbye and says, "Man, you're hard as a rock!"

"Call me Gibraltar," I'll say. "Jib for short."

THE MR. SUN PART

Mr. Sun is your friend. He is generous with Vitamin D, which is essential for your health. Indeed, Vitamin D deficiency was one of the big factors in people getting hammered by Covid.

I know that was true for me. After I got the WuFlu and recovered, I was shocked to learn (through a blood test) that my Vitamin D level was way below the baseline. Experts place the ideal level between 40 and 80 nanograms per milliliter (ng/mL) with levels below 20 ng/mL considered deficient. I was at 19 ng/mL.

And I figured out why.

I grew up in sunny Southern California and baked my skin many a summer at the beach. When the effects began showing on my Scots-Irish face, my dermatologist gave me a lecture on the dangers of sun exposure.

So I went the other way, staying out of the sun as much as possible. I wore a big floppy hat and slathered on the sunscreen.

That's why I had so little Vitamin D in me. While a D

supplement can help a little, it's nothing compared to the D you get from Mr. Sun.

I started spending ten to fifteen minutes outside (this a benefit of living in L.A...maybe the only one left!) I let my torso and legs get the sun, keeping a wide-brimmed hat to protect my face.

That did it. The next time I took a blood test my D level was 34 ng/mL. Nice!

The time after that it was 42 ng/mL. I was golden! (And my bod was a golden-brown).

Here are some tips on getting good D from the sun.

- Wear a bathing suit. Get your torso and legs both involved.
- Get your sun between 11 and 1. Studies have shown this is the optimal time. One study showed that later afternoon sun carries the risk of developing cutaneous malignant melanoma (CCM).
- Aim for 10 - 15 minutes. Don't use sunscreen. You won't burn.
- Wear a brimmed hat and shades if you need to. My face is off limits to Mr. Sun due to the mess I made of it when I was young.
- If you live in a place that gets little sun in the winter months, take a supplement. The recommended daily amount of vitamin D is 400 international units (IU) for children up to age 12, 600 IU for people ages 1 to 70, and 800 IU for people over 70. A calcium-magnesium supplement helps to increase absorption.

THE BOTTOM LINE PART

To put this in simplest terms, I lost 40 pounds, and continue to stay there, by doing this:

- Eat fewer than 60 grams of carbs a day (fruit and veggies don't count).
- Enjoy a civilized cocktail in the evening.
- Have a glass of red with my steaks
- Do some 30-second workouts each day—except Sunday.
- Do some 30-second strength exercises—except Sunday.
- Do an intermittent fast a couple of days out of the week.

If I occasionally don't have a "perfect" day I forget about it, and go on to the next day.

MY IDEAL DAY

I wake up while it is still dark, after six hours of sleep. I drink a small glass of water and pour a fresh cup of coffee from my timed brewer.

I sit in a chair by the window in my living room. If I can see the moon, I give it a nice, lingering look. I listen for the birds to start singing. I enjoy the quiet. (If you're an apartment or city dweller, and noise is a factor, noise-cancelling headphones and soft music or ocean sounds will do the trick.)

I read a Psalm from the Bible, then turn to one of the books in my to-be-read pile. At all costs I avoid the phone, emails, social media, and videos. Reading is healthier than all of these.

My wife joins me for coffee, and we talk a little, and have some prayer time.

I'll eat some breakfast unless I'm doing a partial fast—waiting 16 hours from my meal the night before. I usually do eggs and toast (or tortilla) or oatmeal or, on occasion, cold cereal.

Then I'm into the work part of the day. I write, and the most creative time for my brain is morning.

At some point in the late morning I'll get some sun (one of the benefits of living in Southern Cal), do my 30-minute workouts and strength training.

For a mid-morning snack, an apple, orange, or pepperoni slices and cheese, or nuts (especially cashews). Or all the above!

Lunch is whatever I want it to be. A chicken Caesar salad is nice, or tuna salad wrapped in lettuce. Hamburger patty. But I'll sometimes have a sammie, with sliced beef from a steak the night before, or the occasional pastrami on rye. There are many alternatives to choose from.

I tend to business in the afternoon, including emails and stuff like that.

Mid-afternoon snack celery sticks with peanut butter, or trail mix.

Three o'clock is the beginning of my zombie time. My brain wants to rest. I help it along with a power nap—twenty minutes (an alternative is to lie on my back with my feet up on the bed so the blood comes downward. I relax this way, listening to ocean sounds, for about ten minutes. It really recharges the brain).

I'll do some reading for an hour or so.

Around four o'clock is cocktail time, usually a bourbon rocks or civilized martini.

Then dinner, using the principles described in this book. Once again, my absolute favorite is a rib-eye steak. But other cuts are welcome. My wife makes an outstanding chuck roast in a dutch oven. We'll have a glass of red wine with these.

In the evening, my wife and I take in some viewing. We enjoy old movies the most, especially classic film noir.

My secret sauce in all of this is a great wife. Been married over forty years. Sharing my life with Mrs. C is the absolute best thing for my health and happiness.

I've kept my weight down for almost two years this way.

May it be the same for you. I wish you a good, long, happy life.

Your friend,

Cade

Many thanks for reading my book. If you enjoyed it, please consider leaving a review on Amazon. If this is the ebook version, you can do so by going **here**.

ENDNOTES

1. WHAT WE ALL THOUGHT WAS TRUE IS NOT

1. https://www.prageru.com/video/how-the-government-made-you-fat
2. https://www.ncbi.nlm.nih.gov/pmc/articles/PMC5986484/

3. THE BEEF PART

1. https://www.webmd.com/diet/health-benefits-beef

4. THE BUTTER PART

1. https://www.webmd.com/diet/health-benefits-butter

5. THE BORDEAUX PART

1. https://youtu.be/njm1LkXP2sg

6. THE EXERCISE AND MUSCLE PART (WHICH YOU'LL LOVE)

1. https://www.pennmedicine.org/news/news-blog/2018/march/the-workout-debate-experts-weigh-in-on-cardio-vs-hiit

ABOUT THE AUTHOR

Cade Connors is the pen name of a lawyer and writer who lives near the Pacific Ocean.

www.ingramcontent.com/pod-product-compliance
Lightning Source LLC
LaVergne TN
LVHW052106160826
845678LV00015B/3385

9798366660501